AROMATHERAPY

for Healthy Legs and Feet

by Christine Westwood

Amberwood Publishing Ltd
Park Corner, Park Horsley, East Horsley, Surrey KT24 5RZ
Telephone: 01483 285919

ISBN 1-899308-02-4

Cover design by Clive Holmes Studios

Typeset and designed by
Word Perfect, Christchurch, Dorset.

Printed in Great Britain

CONTENTS

Page No

FOREWORD

Note to Reader

Foreword

Healthy legs and feet are vital to a healthy body and general well-being. If the legs or feet are in poor condition this will often translate to the rest of the body and cause further problems elsewhere. For example, if the arches of the feet are not properly performing their function as shock absorbers, lower back pain and headaches may result. Thus it is very important to take good care of your legs and feet.

Aromatherapy for Healthy Legs and Feet takes an important step towards the abolition of many ailments by familiarising the reader with the structure of the foot and leg, and the causes, symptoms and treatment of many common problems. The serious consequences of improper fitting of shoes and the need for regular foot and leg care are highlighted.

The use of Aromatherapy on both the legs and the feet can have great effect, not only in these areas but also on the whole well-being of the body. Using Essential Oils for bathing and Aromatherapy massage helps to keep legs and feet problem free and in good condition. In my role as a Chiropodist, I am constantly advocating that prevention is far better than cure and that it is never too late to start looking after your feet!

This book, I feel, combines the knowledge and practical guidance necessary for everyone safely to enjoy the pleasures and benefits of Aromatherapy foot and leg care in their own home. I would be happy to recommend Aromatherapy for Healthy Legs and Feet to anyone experiencing problems with their legs and feet, and indeed to anyone wishing to improve their general health.

KIMBY OSBORNE S.L.Ch. M.Inst.Ch.
Training Manager of Scholl Consumer Products

About the Author

Christine Westwood has her own Aromatherapy practice in London where, over the last 10 years, she has developed a synthesis of holistic healing methods called Meta-Aromatherapy. This combines her expertise in Aromatherapy, Art Therapy, Nutrition, Reiki, Counselling, Hypnotherapy and Stress Management.

Christine's involvement in natural healing with plants began in 1982 whilst she was working in the herbal apothecary at the Findhorn Foundation in Scotland. She then trained with Robert Tisserand and became a Founder Director of the Tisserand Aromatherapy Institute. Prior to this, Christine was able to research and develop stress management techniques whilst working as a qualified accountant in the City of London.

Christine's wisdom and wide experience are now being offered to teach others. As well as consultations, her organisation, Christine Westwood Training, has developed a broad spectrum of training programmes which focus on Aromatherapy, Stress Management and Practitioner Care, ranging from informal introductory sessions to a Master's Degree.

This is Christine's third book on Aromatherapy, following the success of her first two titles: *Aromatherapy - A Guide For Home Use* and *Aromatherapy Stress Management - A Guide For Home Use*. She is also a frequent contributor to the media.

Christine enjoys writing and would like to express her thanks to all those involved in the creation of this book. She hopes readers will benefit from her knowledge and discover the healing potential of Essential Oils for themselves.

For further information, write to Christine Westwood Training care of 25 Kite House, The Falcons, Grant Road, London SW11 2NJ.

1 | Aromatherapy Foot and Leg Quiz

Fill in this quiz to identify conditions which can be helped by Aromatherapy for Healthy Legs and Feet.

Do you suffer from cold feet in winter?. . . . . ☐
Do your feet perspire excessively?. . . . . ☐
Are you uncertain of the correct way to cut toenails? . . . . ☐
Do you stand on your feet continuously for more than an hour at a time?. . . . . ☐
Do you suffer from aching feet more than once a week?. . . . . ☐
Do your feet ache even when you are sitting?. . . . . ☐
Do your feet ever feel as if they burn?. . . . . ☐
Do your feet swell: regularly? ☐   only when hot? ☐   rarely? . . . . . . ☐
Do cuts, bruises or insect bites on your feet take a long time to heal? . . . . ☐
Do you suffer from pain in your heels? . . . . ☐
Do you have high arches or low (fallen) arches? . . . . ☐
Do you use an arch support or other foot support? . . . . ☐
Do your shoes rub or feel uncomfortable (e.g. toes tight, heels loose)? . . . . ☐
Do you tend to suffer from any fungal infections (e.g. athlete's foot)? . . . . ☐
Do you suffer from: corns? ☐   callouses? ☐   bunions? . . . . ☐
Are your toenails split even where there has been no injury?. . . . . ☐
Do your toenails have white marks on them where there has been no injury?. . . . . . . ☐
Are you generally sensitive to: man-made fibres? ☐   other materials?. . . . . . ☐
Do you have any rashes on your feet or do you suffer from any allergies? . . . . ☐
Do you suffer from varicose veins or ulcers on your legs? . . . . ☐
Have you lost or gained more than a stone (14 pounds) in weight recently? . . . . ☐
Do you suffer from arteriosclerosis, diabetes or arthritis? . . . . ☐
Do you suffer from problems in your hips, knees, back, head or neck? . . . . ☐
Do you suffer from cramp in your calf muscles? . . . . ☐
Do you tend not to warm up before exercise?. . . . . ☐
Do you tend to avoid a minimum 20 minute walk/exercise 3 times a week? . . . . ☐
Do you jog on hard surfaces (concrete, brick, asphalt) rather than soft
surfaces such as cinder track, grass or sand? . . . . ☐
Do you avoid walking barefoot when there is the opportunity to do so?. . . . . ☐
Have you seen a chiropodist or had specialist foot care in the last year? . . . . ☐
Have your feet never/rarely received massage? ☐   pedicure? ☐   relaxing footbaths? ☐

2 | A Trip Around the Foot

Your feet form the base from which you view your world. Healthy feet predispose you to physical, emotional and mental well-being in the rest of your body: it could be said they enable you to stand on your own two feet!

Taking care of your feet, then, is important. Attention is frequently paid to headaches, backache, colds, stomach upsets, etc., but very few people are aware of how many of these ailments are directly influenced by lack of adequate foot care. For example, a headache or backache may be directly linked to fallen arches.

Diseased or damaged feet can have a profound effect on your lifestyle, making you irritable (perhaps complaining that your feet are killing you!), affecting your concentration and, in severe cases, confining you to your home or necessitating an operation.

A sound maxim is: "If you look after your feet, you look after yourself."

So now is the time to discover what is a foot! There are fascinating facts about your feet which, in combination with Aromatherapy Foot Care, will enable you to reap the benefits of caring for them.

Let's start from inside the foot and work our way outwards.

Did you know that each of your feet contains 26 bones? Where the bones of your feet meet they form joints. The different ways in which the bones join together determine the kind of joint which is formed. A ball and socket joint, for example the **hip joint**, permits movement in all directions. A condyloid joint is very similar, allowing all movements except twisting: try twisting your **toes**! Hinge joints, such as the **knee**, will only move up or down; and gliding joints,such as are found in the **tarsal** area of the foot, allow the bones to glide over each other for very short distances.

Binding your bones together at the joints are **ligaments**. These are strong bands of fibrous tissue which enable movement but at the same time restrict extreme movement. Ligaments help to maintain the **arches** and the tendons at the front of your feet.

The muscles in your feet and legs are mainly voluntary muscles. This means they are under the control of your will: you direct them and they provide the power you need to move. Since your muscles only work when they are contracting, they can pull but cannot push, and for this reason the muscles are usually arranged in pairs so that as one muscle contracts, the other lengthens. The muscles are attached to your bones by tendons; for example, the **Achilles tendon**.

Your feet also contain a number of important arches whose main function is to act as shock absorbers. The main arch runs along the length of the inner side of your feet and is called the **inner longitudinal arch**. It is from this arch that most of the springing action of your feet arises. (This is the main area affected if a person becomes flat-footed.) Another important arch is located at the ball of your feet, forming a dome-like pad which is increased through barefoot walking. Practically all pain in the ball of the foot is due to weakness in this arch. Along the side of your foot lies the **outer longitudinal arch**, which contacts the ground when weight is placed upon your foot. Finally, there is a minor arch called the **transverse arch** which runs across the foot.

These are all enclosed within your skin: a waterproof, flexible, and elastic covering which protects your body from infection and the harmful rays of the sun. The inner layer, or dermis, contains the blood vessels and nerve endings (which react to pressure, pain and temperature), the sweat glands (which remove waste products and regulate your body temperature), and the hair follicles. The epidermis is the outermost protective layer which is thickest on the soles of your feet and palms. Other functions of the skin are respiration and absorption, for example, of Essential Oils and vitamin D from sunlight.

Nails protect your fingers and toes, acting as tools or weapons! Only part of the nail is alive: the base (matrix), which, if damaged by injury or disease, often results in deformity of the nail. The cuticle grows over this base. Underneath the nail is the nail bed – the large area of pink skin which plays an important part in the nutrition of the nail itself. It takes from 10 to 18 months for the toenails to re-grow completely: twice as long as your fingernails. Nails grow faster in summer than in winter, in younger people and during pregnancy.

Now that we have completed our trip around the foot, let's follow a day in the life of your legs and feet!

3 | The Miracle of Movement

So what happens to your feet and legs as you go about your day?

Did your know that you are always taller first thing in the morning? This is due to your backbone stretching out while you sleep and the absence of gravity compressing your spine. Once upright, gravity affects your whole body; for example, it weakens the muscles which cover your abdomen. These are normally relaxed, but on standing produce a contraction which, from your twenties onwards, functions less efficiently. Rare are the adults who can stand sideways in front of a mirror and breathe outwards without noticing the "potbelly" effect.

Did you know that your head shrinks when you stand due to gravity draining the blood from it, whilst your legs swell in volume for the same reason?

As you stand, the heat given off by your body rises steadily upwards, surrounding you in a current of warm air, which is half an inch thick at the ankles but widens to eight inches around the head. This rising hot air transports what we call household dust, 80 percent of which is dead skin cells. Clothes can impede the process of exfoliating dead skin, so choose natural fibres which allow your skin to breathe, and change your footwear and hosiery regularly to benefit the well-being of your whole body.

So, now you have managed to stand – which incidentally requires the co-ordination of over 200 muscles – it is time to take a step forward, but it's not as easy as you might think! Walking is an inherently unsteady movement, involving the attempt to balance first on one leg, then the other – without falling over – which is quite remarkable, considering the size of your feet in relation to your body.

A number of movements in the rest of your body occur as you walk. Some of these are minute: for example, the cheeks of your face flap; your eyes bounce up and down in their sockets with each step, along with your internal organs, such as the stomach, kidneys, liver and heart. Your head and ears gently wiggle, your arms sway – in fact, your whole body is in motion.

Just getting one leg to lift takes over 40 muscles working together. As this movement works its way through your body, your back muscles are needed quickly to return your chest and shoulders to an upright stance. However, this backward movement of your abdomen, chest and head would result in your falling down on your buttocks if it were not for another series of muscles in your abdomen pulling you upright. Turning sideways involves muscles in your stomach, hips and chest as well as the long muscle of your outer thigh which is one of the strongest in your body.

Now you have managed to stand and move your legs, it's time to use your feet! As your feet move forward, just before your heel contacts the ground it relaxes, which allows it to absorb the resulting impact. The bones in the front of your feet are now faced with the same impact and, loosening up, embed themselves in the soft tissue on the soles of your feet. A brief moment later your legs are ready for take-off again, so your bones snap together into the tightest formation possible, creating an instant rod-like lever to propel your body forward.

Around most contracting muscles and moving joints are sensors which send electrical impulses to your brain. These change with each movement; for example, the patterns produced during running never happen in any other movement. Your brain receptors keep track of these movements, usually without you realising it. For example, as you straighten your ankle whilst getting out of a chair, you do not need to keep looking down to check your ankle. As you turn your body, your bones are protected by finely-moulded sacs of lubricating fluid, which again you are unaware of unless illness, knocks, or general tiredness cause swelling, and your body aches. Balanced exercise, relaxation and care with Essential Oils can prevent the occurrence of many problems.

All these movements are choreographed by your brain, which receives the signals through nerve fibres, registering that movement has commenced. Whilst you are active the signals continue, but will stop while you are at rest unless confused by the motion of travelling, for example, whilst at sea. Nausea can result due to the bombardment of feedback from your brain, confused by the constantly changing landscape into thinking that it is your body which is moving and not the sea.

Those of you who are more active may be interested to know the processes required for jogging and running and their effect on your body. Sir Roger Bannister, the Oxford researcher who ran the first sub-four minute mile in 1954, based his research on the premise that no muscle can move unless it has the necessary burst of energy. He observed that there were three main stages as the muscles responded. One of the chemical processes in your body triggers the flares of energy (called ATP) within muscle cells that enable you to move. This process is important for those emergencies, like rushing for your train, but not for longer distances. This is why sprinters have not managed to reduce their time, whilst long distance runners have, thanks to more efficient use of the following process.

The blood sugar levels now adjust to recharge the flares, which have expended heat and pumped the thighs so tight as to block most of the ordinary blood flow. Blood-sugar is then released from stored energy as you start jogging. This is the main reason for loosening up before a run, apart from the possibility of pulling a muscle. In addition, actually thinking about movement, before commencing an activity, triggers your body's reaction to begin releasing this energy. After about two minutes of activity, lactic acid is produced (rather like a milky liquid), which stays in the muscles and stops the ATP from recharging. It is this which produces the common feeling of sudden tiredness whilst exercising.

However, it is the third process that most runners enjoy, which is often referred to as 'a second wind'. Fresh oxygen then pours into the tiring muscles and then the blood sugar recharges the ATP without the lactic acid and makes carbohydrates, fats and proteins available to fuel the muscles.

The deep breathing induced by running promotes the circulation of blood around your bones, which is where your white blood cells are produced. These help your body fight disease, so an increase in antibodies, due to increased muscle activity, may explain the common report of fewer colds experienced by runners. It also has an effect on the renewal of bone tissue, encouraging its growth.

4 | A Firm Foundation

It has been estimated that on average people cover 70,000 miles on their feet in a lifetime, which equates to around 18,000 steps each day. Over 14 million people a year seek medical advice for foot and leg ailments, many of which can be connected to poor posture and bad circulation. It is questionable whether pain and stiffness arise because an organ is diseased, or whether they are created by poor posture and a lack of exercise which has led to the malfunction of the associated organ.

The foundation of your body, at your feet, can be likened to the foundation of a house. If the structure is not carefully in place, eventually the walls will crack and problems ensue. Once your feet are out of balance, so is your body. As a famous song suggests, your feet and your entire body are articulated with one bone connecting to another. All posture starts with your feet; for example, if your feet turn out, then your legs will also turn out and great stress is placed on the supporting bones and muscles. The surfaces where one bone meets another can become irritated, which can manifest in knee, hip, lower back, neck and head pains.

So what is the best way to stand or move on your feet? When you walk, your feet are not rigid levers moving your body forward. They firstly make contact with the back outer section of your heels and then move forward along the outer edge onto the balls of your feet, pushing off with the big toes. You can tell whether or not you have been walking properly by examining the heels of your shoes. Your shoes should be worn down at the back of your heel, and slightly to the outside.

Although facing straight ahead, your feet do not always move in a straight line. If you traced the movement, it would look like a curving line, shifting the body from side to side. In the past, our ancestors swung by their arms from branch to branch, and perhaps it is this that is continued today in our swaying walk! So, are humans designed for standing, or is it a feat to which our bodies are still becoming acclimatised? Humans are unique in their upright stance, as even those animals who do manage to stand are forced back on all fours in seconds through the pain which standing causes. Humans are different: the curving backwards of the bottom few bones in your spine creates a spring, which allows turning and balancing and enables you to walk.

Are You Flexible?

Both adults and children can benefit from foot and leg massage using Essential Oils, along with gentle stretching. As you grow older, without care your ligaments become less flexible, shortening and tightening, resulting in stiffness and less mobility. To test your mobility, try this out. Without straining, see if you can touch your toes: a child can do this easily. A flexible person can sit with his/her back straight and legs stretched out at a 90-degree angle without pain. Check how flexible your upper spine and neck are by trying the following movement: do not force it; sit in a straight-backed chair with your hips touching the back of the seat, your arms loose, and hands holding the seat near the rear of your chair. You should be able to turn your head to the left or right with your chin parallel to your shoulders. If you feel pain with this movement, it indicates tightness in your ligaments. If, in the same position, with your chin stretched forward, your head can drop to the right or to the left, and your ear touches your shoulder without pain, this indicates mobility of your lower ligaments. The ligaments in the back of the legs can be tested by bending forward in a bow with your head and arms dropping loosely.

People over 30 years of age who lead a sedentary life and have poor posture will often feel a degree of tightening and may experience pain in their feet along with common ailments such as headaches and backaches. Ligaments may also tighten due to sudden chills, arthritis and gout, or strain from lifting heavy weights and awkwardly twisting your body. You may not feel any pain immediately, but the resulting stiffness and rigidity can mean that any movement of the ligament becomes painful. However, a lack of movement will exacerbate the condition. A gentle, progressive programme of exercise should help free the compressed nerves which are causing the pain. If in any doubt, seek medical attention.

5 | Preventative Footcare

Long before you are born, while you are still in your mother's womb, the bones in your feet begin to form. This process continues right up to 25 years of age. Therefore, it is most important to look after feet in these vital early years.

Young Feet and Preventative Care

Western society encourages us to cover up babies' feet at the earliest opportunity with cute booties or socks and tiny shoes. If you watch babies, they spend a lot of their time flexing and bending their fingers and toes, and this unhindered movement is an important part of their muscle development. As soon as their feet are covered, their movement is restricted. Ideally, children would be allowed to go barefoot until six or seven, permitting full mobility of their growing foot muscles and thus contributing to their overall health. However, feet do need the protection of footwear on concrete and other hard surfaces.

Footwear should be flexible and have plenty of room in which feet can flex and extend. Sandals are ideal, but take care when drying them to avoid cracking the leather, as this can cause blisters, sores, or even warts where it rubs. Plimsolls (not trainers!) are the next best choice for children, as their feet can breathe through the canvas. Care must be taken to avoid fungal infections which are encouraged by the rubber sole, especially in hot weather: it is best to have several pairs and alternate them.

Teenagers have quite comfortable and sensible footwear now that boots and flat shoes are the fashion but, typically in adulthood, fashion encourages women to wear high heels, which throw the whole body out of alignment and can cause backache as a result of strain on the thighs and legs. Constant wearing of high heels can lead to tendons at the front of the feet becoming stretched, whilst the Achilles tendon shortens, resulting in aches and cramps. A more liberated fashion for healthy feet would be the avoidance of high heels for life. Narrow and tapered shoes encourage overlapping toes, ingrowing toenails, inflammation and bunions.

The increase in sports activity and the resulting wearing of trainers has been positive in terms of overall health and general foot care, but brings with it potential foot odour, Athlete's Foot and verrucae.

Choosing Footwear

Choosing shoes for healthy feet can be quite a challenge. Properly fitted shoes should allow a space of one-quarter of an inch beyond the big toe when standing.

The widest part of the shoe should match the width of the foot, the shoe following the natural outline of the foot, fitting snugly yet not too tightly. The back of the heel should both fit and be flexible, keeping the shoe in place, but without being tight. The heel should form a solid base and ideally be no more than a quarter of an inch high. The front of your shoes should be suited to your foot shape, their depth allowing space for your toes, and they should be made of material that can breathe, e.g. canvas or soft leather.

Choose a shoe for its fit, that is the shape, width and depth that best suits your foot, considering thickness of sole, narrowness of heel and amount of arch. Look for good workmanship: a shoe should feel right when you try it on and not need breaking in. Socks should not be too tight as these, too, can cause skin irritation, resulting in blisters, corns and callouses.

It is important to wear shoes which are appropriate to the activity for which they are designed. Running shoes, for example, are designed for movement in a straight line and give different support from high-impact sports shoes such as those for jogging, squash or aerobics, where stress can cause problems with the knees, shins and ankles.

If you are pregnant or very overweight, adjustable shoes with low heels are advisable. These support the extra weight and unbalanced posture, avoiding swollen feet, painful ankles and varicose veins, whilst minimising fatigue.

Specially made moulded shoes can be a great aid for painful and uncomfortable foot conditions. They are prepared from plaster of Paris or, more helpfully, a dynamic mould of cork and slow-setting plastic which forms as the person walks around until the mould is set. They do not cure the condition but do allow people to stay on their feet longer without becoming tired. The disadvantages are that such shoes are usually not very attractive and can cost up to four or five times more than ordinary shoes.

The Benefit of Exercise and Movement

If we liken the heart and veins to a stream, its life forms nourished by the fresh water as it flows through, you can appreciate that if there is no current in the stream, it becomes stagnant and all kinds of algae develop. Your heart, similarly, receives its nourishment from your blood supply, which is maintained through regular exercise whilst you are young and through keeping mobile and active as you get older. If you do not exercise, your veins become furred up and the blood supply does not flow so readily.

You need to exercise your feet, too, in order to keep them in good shape. The tendons and muscles that hold the bones of your feet together require gentle exercise to become flexible yet strong. Exercise will not wear them out! However, people are sometimes over-enthusiastic when they start exercising. This, too, may cause problems since the muscles will ache unless there is a slow and steady build up of strength. At this point people often give up, so begin gradually on a suitable surface such as grass, with the appropriate shoes and, above all, warm up your muscles first by stretching, bending and rotating your feet and legs. Choose exercise which you enjoy, whether it is walking, running, playing tennis, swimming, yoga or another activity. As your body becomes accustomed to exercise you can gradually increase the time without undue strain, and the range of exercise can be extended so that your heart increases its capacity.

Ageing Feet

As you grow older, your feet age too. The heart finds it harder to pump blood to your feet and so the skin and underlying tissues suffer. It is best to avoid constricting the blood vessels by crossing your legs, wearing tight socks or smoking, which are all detrimental to your circulation. Ageing feet are more susceptible to corns, callouses, bunions and hammer toes – all the result of poor footwear, although some conditions have an hereditary factor. Avoid irritation and infection from such sources as cuts, sunburn, hot water bottles, ill-fitting shoes, socks with holes and darns. Wear clean hosiery each day and do not try to deal with these conditions yourself using unsterilised implements. Take care with your diet to provide the vitamins and minerals needed through good quality food, with supplements as necessary. Simple foot exercises, which can be done sitting in a chair, are also beneficial.

6 | Foot and Leg Conditions and Aromatherapy Treatment

Check the condition of your feet regularly. They frequently receive no attention until pain prompts action. There are a number of minor problems which, if left unattended, may develop into more serious and permanent conditions. Aromatherapy, using pure essential oils, is useful for many of these conditions, so check this section and the Essential Oils Guide for the appropriate oils to use as well as the methods section, "Aromatherapeutics", for directions on how to use them. There are also ready-made 'recipes' for you to try in the Aromatherapy Blends section. If in any doubt consult your GP, who may suggest that you visit a chiropodist or use specialist proprietary foot aids.

Dry Skin and Abrasions

One of the first conditions to pay attention to is areas of dry skin. Similarly, if your skin is rubbed continually as a result of tight footwear it may not hurt initially, but will later form a protection of hard skin. If unattended, infection may follow and develop into some of the conditions listed below.

TREATMENT FOR DRY SKIN, ABRASIONS

Daily bathing with Essential Oil Foot Baths and Aromatherapy Foot Massage.
Shins and knees can also become dry as the skin is thinner over these areas. Have daily Essential Oil Baths and use Aromatherapy Leg Massage.

Skin Conditions and Allergies

An allergy is an individual's reaction to an environment or a substance which is well tolerated in the normal course of events. Generally, an allergic reaction will be experienced when the immune system is depleted, for example when you are feeling run down. A common cause of allergies is found in the materials making up your shoes, whether synthetic or natural. Rashes may develop over a period of time where the shoe material and the foot make contact.

Common allergens are: synthetic fibres or washing powder; metals (often precipitated by a reaction to having pierced ears); chemicals used in shoe production (formaldehyde, copper sulphate, coal tar derivatives etc.); rubber shoe components; cements, which are used to line the heel pads; or the tanning compounds used in treating leather.

Care must be taken to ensure that pure quality Essential Oils are used for treatments. Although it is pleasant to have soaps, lotions and perfumes fragranced synthetically, they have no therapeutic value and may indeed contain allergens themselves.

TREATMENT FOR SKIN CONDITIONS AND ALLERGIES

Avoid excessive perspiration. It is helpful to try to identify and avoid the source of the reaction by changing your footwear frequently and noting any improvement. For example, those who discover they are allergic to nylon may find they benefit from wearing pure cotton, silk or wool.

Essential Oil Foot Baths and, once any rashes have subsided and broken skin has healed, Aromatherapy Foot Massage.

Essential Oils work to strengthen the body's various systems, thus improving the immune system. If conditions persist, seek medical attention.

Corns, Bursitis, Callouses and Bunions

Corns are painful, cone-shaped overgrowths of horny skin on the toe joints, mainly caused by the repeated friction and pressure of ill-fitting shoes. Irritation and pressure are exacerbated when toes continually rub against each other inside tapered shoes.

There are several different types of corn: hard corn, the most common, found on any part of the foot; soft corn, which is white and rubbery and occurs only between the toes where perspiration collects; seed corn, found mostly on the sole of the foot, usually in multiples, and gives the sensation of walking on grit.

An interesting aspect of corns is their ability to forecast the weather: a drop in atmospheric pressure is signalled by increased pain in the corn.

Bursitis is created when a bursa (a small fluid-filled sac lubricating the joints) becomes inflamed. The area is then surrounded by a ring of inflamed skin. A bursa may be located on either side of the Achilles tendon or under the heel (e.g. if shoes rub) but is most commonly found on a bunion or enlarged joint.

Callouses are similar to corns, but without the regular round shape or smooth central eye. A burning pain due to pressure from hard skin on a large number of nerve endings arises, along with thickening skin on the soles. Callouses can form on the side of the nails as a natural defence against ingrowing toenails, but in general they are caused by friction and pressure from shoes.

Bunions are a common foot condition. When mild there is usually no pain, but incorrectly-shaped or badly-fitted shoes will put pressure on the joint. As the condition worsens, a thickening of the joint (exostosis) occurs and then a bursa forms to protect the joint. As the bursa in turn becomes inflamed, a bunion forms to protect it.

Bunions are thought to be largely hereditary. However, consideration should be given to contributory factors such as the influence of family lifestyle. For example, your diet and exercise regimes since childhood will affect the functioning of your internal organs, skin and posture, and thus the condition of your feet. Often these habits – even the way you walk – are copied from your elders.

TREATMENT FOR CORNS

Corns are best treated by chiropody or specialised proprietary products and avoiding ill-fitting shoes. Aromatherapy can be used as a preventative measure, keeping skin soft and supple.

Essential Oil Foot Baths and Aromatherapy Massage are indicated.

To treat callouses, soak your feet in an Aromatherapy Foot Bath and use a pumice stone or a proprietary foot file. Take care not to break the skin, particularly if you are diabetic, as broken skin may result in infection.

For bunions, avoid tight-fitting shoes, high heels and becoming very obese. Visit a chiropodist, who may recommend a proprietary aid, special shoes or minor surgery in chronic cases.

Chilblains and Circulatory Diseases

Chilblains are due to bad circulation and are often associated with cold, damp conditions. They are generally found on the hands and feet, but can affect any of the extremities, including the nose and ears. The skin looks taut and shiny, is dark red or purple in colour, itchy and tender, and may be swollen. Tight footwear worsens the condition by restricting the circulation.

Circulatory diseases can cause difficulty in walking, pain in the feet (sometimes hurting even while at rest), varicose veins, tightness in the calf, regular cramping or coldness, discomfort and swelling. The body is then unable to supply enough blood to the legs, and exercise causes sharp pain in the muscles. It can even result in going lame. It is wise to check any indicated vascular problems.

TREATMENT FOR CHILBLAINS AND CIRCULATORY DISEASES

Essential Oil Foot Baths should be used in the first instance to heal any broken skin. Hot and cold Essential Oil Foot Baths, finishing with warm water, aid the circulation. Once the skin is healed, or if there is no broken skin, daily Aromatherapy Foot and Leg Massage is indicated. Your feet should be kept warm at all times, using thermal footwear if necessary.

Essential Oil Baths and full body Aromatherapy Massage help generally to improve the circulation.

Consult your chiropodist or doctor if blisters or irritations do not heal readily.

Arthritis and Gout

Arthritis is an acute or chronic condition which affects the joints and muscles, creating inflammation and pain. This can be aggravated by stress, injury or a poor diet inducing high acid/alkaline levels. Of the various forms of arthritis – rheumatoid, stress-induced, infection-related, and osteo-arthritis – it is normally the latter which manifests itself in the feet. The cartilage degenerates and the bones become distorted and waste away; the linings of the joints become swollen and full of fluid, retarding their movement; the muscles are then unable to function effectively and they too begin to waste away. Flexing toes is then painful, with the result that walking becomes difficult.

Gout is a disease which may attack any joint in the body and is thought to be related to arthritis. Most arthritis sufferers are women but most gout victims are men. The majority of sufferers are over 30 years old. Possibly inherited, and linked to hormonal change as women tend not to get gout until after the menopause, gout upsets the balance of purine contained in the blood. Joints then become painful, swollen, hot and tender, with reddening of the skin, which may even turn purple, along with irritation of the nerve endings.

TREATMENT FOR ARTHRITIS AND GOUT

Aromatherapy Massage helps to maintain mobility of the muscles and joints and also to balance the emotions, as arthritis has been linked to a person's emotional state.

Take frequent Essential Oil Baths and Aromatherapy Massage.

Seek medical attention if necessary.

Fungal/Viral Infection: Nails, Warts, Verrucae and Athlete's Foot

Nails

Fungal infections are often confused with other conditions such as psoriasis, contact dermatitis and sensitivity to footwear. They frequently arise from blisters which have caused sores, providing a fertile environment in the irritated skin for the growth of fungus.

Fungal nail infection is a very common condition where the nail is infected by fungus in a similar manner to the way skin is infected by athlete's foot. The infection can be so mild as to be undetectable to the eye.

Warts (Verrucae)

A wart on the foot is technically known as a verruca. This looks similar to a corn but is infectious and is normally found on the sole of the foot, yet rarely on a pressure point. The wart stands out from the surrounding tissue and contains little black dots (blood vessels). It usually hurts when squeezed and can occur singly or in multiples. Children are more susceptible than adults, girls more so than boys. Verrucae may be contracted in communal changing areas if your skin is cut or irritated, so care should be taken under these conditions.

PREVENTION AND TREATMENT OF WARTS

A chiropodist may treat warts with acid paste or liquid, electric current, freezing or by surgery. Verrucae may also respond to suggestion: it has been noted that often they disappear between an initial examination and the time set for their removal.

Essential Oil Baths, Aromatherapy Foot Massage and foot hygiene are of paramount importance for viral conditions. Essential Oils of Tea Tree and Lemon may be applied neat to the wart using a cotton bud, twice a day, after bathing.

Athlete 's Foot

Athlete's Foot is usually found between the fourth and fifth toes but it can spread to all of the toes and to the top and soles of the feet as well. There are three types: wet and oozing, inflamed and scaly. The affected skin appears white and macerated with peeling or red and inflamed skin. It itches and is tender and sore blisters may form. Known also as Bombay Foot Rot or Golfer's Itch, the condition is often thought to arise through walking barefoot in communal bathing areas such as swimming pools.

PREVENTION AND TREATMENT OF ATHLETE'S FOOT

Avoid walking barefoot in communal changing areas. Use clean towels. For a fungal nail infection, visit the chiropodist.

Athlete's Foot can normally be cleared up by consistent application of a few drops of neat Essential Oil of Tea Tree to the affected area, using a cotton bud.

Perspiration

Did you know that there are 250,000 sweat glands in the feet, typically producing a quarter of an egg-cupful of sweat each day? When the skin's sweat glands produce excessive amounts of perspiration, this can affect the whole body including the feet, which feel damp to the touch. The skin may become white and tender. An offensive odour may be given off due to bacteria acting on the fatty content of the perspiration, causing it to decompose. Malfunction of the sweat glands in the feet can also cause too little perspiration, resulting in dry skin, which can become very thin, flaky, or both. This is more common in elderly people for whom the affected skin becomes sore and splits, and may develop hard corns.

TREATMENT FOR PERSPIRATION

Strict foot hygiene is necessary. Foot Baths with Essential Oils of Cypress and Tea Tree are effective against excessive perspiration. Alternating hot and cold foot baths, ending with cold, are helpful.

Dry skin can be removed with a pumice stone or proprietary file and Aromatherapy Foot Massage is advisable to soften and heal the skin.

Seek advice from a chiropodist if the condition persists.

Foot Odour

Foot odour can be caused by excessive perspiration; a build-up of toxins, often due to poor circulation; or by the tension of muscles held in an unnatural position in badly-fitting shoes.

TREATMENT FOR FOOT ODOUR

Take care with foot hygiene, changing footwear frequently. Aromatherapy Massage will improve the lymphatic and circulatory systems, releasing the build-up of toxins.

Daily Essential Oil Foot Baths and Aromatherapy Foot Massage using Cypress and Rosemary are indicated.

Toenail Conditions

Infected toenails result from a fungal disease where the front of the toenail becomes overgrown, pitted and opaque, with the nail and the skin underneath becoming powdery. The entire nail and those around it can be destroyed if the condition spreads.

For every 10 people who suffer from nail infections, it has been estimated that three have ingrowing toenails. The toenail grows inward and down into the flesh on either side of the nail. The cut and irritated flesh becomes inflamed and infection may ensue, becoming septic if untreated. Usually found on the big toe, the condition is painful (as a sharp part of the nail pushes inwards against the skin) and is most commonly caused by improper nail cutting. Toenails should always be cut straight across. Avoid trimming the nails too short, in too curved a shape or leaving sharp corners. Another cause is ill-fitting shoes and socks.

A ramshorn nail is a comparatively rare condition where the nail becomes deformed into a shape reminiscent of a ram's horn, usually following an injury to the nail root. This results in permanent deformity requiring regular chiropody. Hangnail is a condition where the skin at the side of the nail becomes thick and then splits. To avoid inflammation, cut it away rather than pull it out.

White marks on the nails usually indicate air pockets which arise as the result of injury and will normally grow out with the nail. Nails are more susceptible to injury and splitting when there is a nutritional deficiency.

Brittle nails are more often found in older people, but may also be caused by poor circulation, too much fluoride in drinking water or diabetes.

Thickened nails occur when the nail growth becomes distorted due to an injury or nerve irritation that affects the nail bed, shoe pressure, a fungus infection, circulatory problems or diabetes.

TREATMENT FOR TOENAIL CONDITIONS

Cut and trim toenails carefully. Seek medical attention if the condition becomes severe, or visit a chiropodist.

For infected toenails, use Essential Oils of Tea Tree and Lavender in an Essential Oil Foot Bath.

In mild cases of ingrowing toenails, use Essential Oils such as Frankincense and Lavender to soften the skin and soothe the inflammation in an Essential Oil Foot Bath. Once inflammation has subsided, regular Aromatherapy Foot Massage is helpful.

High Arches and Fallen Arches

A high arched foot is caused by the ligaments and tissues in the sole of the foot becoming contracted, manifesting in an exaggeratedly-high arch. This results in the heel and the ball of the foot alone bearing the weight, causing painful horny pads of skin under the bones of the toes and a pigeon-toed walk. A short Achilles tendon can result in an abnormally high arch. For high arches, high heels may feel more comfortable, especially if you are accustomed to wearing them.

Fallen arches should not be confused with low arches, which may be quite healthy. Indeed, babies and children usually seem flat-footed, due to the layers of fat which cover the arch. A fallen arch is caused by muscles and ligaments becoming strained and stretched so that the arches can no longer function to absorb the shock of each step. Thus the weight of the body is taken by the arch instead of being distributed through the toes and heels.

TREATMENT FOR HIGH AND FALLEN ARCHES

Aromatherapy Foot Massage strengthens foot muscles. Walking barefoot can help fallen arches. However, consult a specialist if you are in pain or having difficulty walking.

Cramps

Cramps are caused by muscle contractions. They can be triggered by heavy sweating, either during hot weather or as a result of participating in an active sport.

TREATMENT FOR CRAMPS

Follow first-aid procedures. If you have been sweating, drinking some water with a pinch of salt will restore the electrolyte balance and relieve the cramp. Stretch the muscles to release the cramp. Firmly pressing the point between the fourth toe and the little toe has been found helpful to release cramp in the leg quickly.

Aromatherapy Foot Massage using Essential Oils of Rosemary and Marjoram will relax the muscles and promote circulation. When used on a regular basis, it has been known to reduce the likelihood of cramps.

Muscular Aches and Pains

Muscular pain as a result of over-exertion responds well to Aromatherapy Massage, following a warm Essential Oil Bath.

Strained Muscles

A strained or pulled muscle may result from an awkward or sudden movement. The injured muscle or tendon then hurts when the person tries to repeat the movement, and stiffness develops. There will also be swelling and discolouration around the site of the injury.

TREATMENT FOR STRAINED MUSCLES

Follow first-aid procedures. Take an Essential Oil Foot Bath and apply an Aromatherapy Compress. Aromatherapy Massage is beneficial once any swelling has reduced.

Sprains

A sprained joint occurs when the ligaments which hold the bones together are over-stretched or torn. A common occurrence, they can be extremely painful. If in any doubt as to whether the bone is fractured or broken, seek medical aid.

TREATMENT FOR SPRAINS

Follow first-aid procedures. Use Essential Oil Foot Baths and an Aromatherapy Compress.

Cellulite

Often referred to as "orange peel skin", this is an unappealing condition, usually bemoaned by women. Contributory factors include constipation; fatigue; lack of exercise; smoking; and an unbalanced diet which includes too much dairy produce, sugar, tea, coffee and/or alcohol. A sluggish circulation and a poorly functioning lymph system exacerbate the condition. The skin appears to be lumpy, dimpled and streaky, which is due to fat deposits formed through the retention of water and toxins. These lodge in the skin, usually around the thighs, hips and buttocks, but may also be found on the upper arms. The skin often feels cold to the touch and painful when pressed. Women are more prone to cellulite at times of hormonal change, such as puberty, pregnancy and the menopause. Cellulite affects thin people as well as the overweight.

TREATMENT FOR CELLULITE

Regular gentle, rhythmic exercise, such as walking and swimming. Avoid overly vigorous exercise.

Dry skin brushing with a natural bristle brush helps cleanse the body of stored toxins by stimulating the circulation and the lymphatic system, encouraging the body to break down any fatty deposits, and removing dead skin cells, which unblocks the pores. Over a period of time the shape and tone of the muscles improve too. In the morning, it provides a stimulating start to your day! Use circular movements starting at your feet and working upwards.

Essential Oil Baths and firm Aromatherapy Full Body Massage, along with Foot and Leg Massage, are helpful.

Essential Oils which encourage the elimination of toxins and excess water are recommended.

Water Retention – Oedema

This condition tends to cause swelling in the ankles, feet and legs, making feet feel cramped in shoes by the end of the day, particularly if there is a lymph infection present. Manifesting primarily around joints, the ankles and knees are particularly susceptible. Fibrous tissue may arise as a result of infection, which should not be left unattended. Oedema or water retention is aggravated by heat and pregnancy.

TREATMENT FOR OEDEMA

Rest with your feet up, preferably keeping them above the level of your head, unless you have been medically advised not to. This allows the fluid to drain away from the ankles and feet. If necessary, you can arrange some pillows at the base of your bed to rest your legs fully as you sleep. If standing or sitting for long periods of time, intersperse this with periods of movement, with help on hand if necessary. Check your diet for excess salt, sugar, tea and coffee, as these aggravate the condition. Even a congenital pre-disposition to oedema can be minimised by careful attention to diet, exercise and lifestyle.

Essential Oil Baths are indicated. A full body Aromatherapy Massage is particularly beneficial for this condition. However, Aromatherapy Foot and Leg Massage alone can be used effectively.

Varicose Veins

These can occur anywhere in the body, but are typically found in the legs. They are caused by weakness of the walls and valves of the veins, leading to blood stagnation. They have a swollen and knotted appearance, frequently causing a nagging pain even when resting. Often associated with standing for long periods, they can also be caused by bad circulation, excess weight, tight clothing, damage to the leg resulting from an injury, or excess cholesterol blocking the arteries. They may also appear during pregnancy. Ulcers can form along the lines of the veins due to pooling of the blood. It is important to improve circulation in order to reverse stagnation and allow oxygenated blood to the area, or the ulcer will not heal. This can be alternated with periods of rest, with the feet raised above hip level. Although typically associated with hereditary weaknesses, careful attention to diet, exercise and lifestyle will reduce the effect of a congenital pre-disposition to varicose veins.

TREATMENT FOR VARICOSE VEINS

Avoid standing still for long periods or sitting with your legs crossed. Put your feet up higher than head level whenever possible. Exercise your calf muscles, flexing your feet up and down and rotating your ankles in both directions.

Where possible, take a gentle daily walk to help your circulation. Never massage over varicose veins. However, Essential Oil Baths and Aromatherapy Compresses are beneficial. It can also be helpful to wear support hosiery.

Seek medical attention if varicose veins are causing persistent problems.

Arteriosclerosis

This occurs when the arteries have thickened so that it is difficult for the blood to flow. Ulcers may also develop which are slow to heal.

TREATMENT FOR ARTERIOSCLEROSIS

Seek medical attention and use Essential Oil Baths and Aromatherapy Compresses.

Bruises

For first-aid purposes, you may apply NEAT Lavender Essential Oil to a bruise, e.g. whilst out walking. At all other times use an Aromatherapy Compress.

Cuts

After bathing the area, Lavender or Tea Tree may be used NEAT for first-aid purposes to reduce the possibility of infection and the likelihood of scarring, and to encourage the skin to heal.

Burns and Sunburn

For minor burns apply first-aid techniques and then you may use NEAT Essential Oil of Lavender. Protect the area from infection if necessary. Sunburn can be soothed and skin renewal encouraged by a tepid bath with Lavender Essential Oil.

Insect Bites and Repellents

Whilst you are exercising outdoors, Essential Oils can help to keep insects such as mosquitoes at bay. Should you get stung or bitten, apply Lavender and Tea Tree immediately. A boon when out in nature, these also work for bramble and nettle stings.

Ringworm

Ringworm forms circles on the skin and may affect the knees. Tea Tree baths and Aromatherapy Massage blends are helpful for this condition. Seek medical advice.

9 | Aromatherapeutics: Methods for Using Essential Oils in Foot and Leg Care

The Aromatherapy Pedicure

The Aromatherapy Pedicure is a suggested weekly procedure. This is especially important if you have a health condition which can affect your feet. Diabetics should ensure that they have regular professional foot care as they may have poor circulation and reduced sensation and so may not be aware of their foot problems.

1. Check for any cuts, abrasions, sores, corns, callouses or infections.
2. Check the length of your toenails and cut as necessary, but not too short, using toenail cutters (remember, always in a straight line to avoid encouraging ingrowing nails).
3. Remove any rough skin with a file or proprietary product. A pumice stone can be used during a foot bath if necessary.
4. Use the Essential Oil Foot Bath Routine and Aromatherapy Foot and Leg Massage which are found later in this chapter.

Aromatherapy Foot Hygiene

The skin is the body's largest organ and it needs to be able to breathe. Air cannot circulate freely whilst your feet are covered, so wear natural fibres next to your skin. Change your footwear regularly and, weather permitting, wear open style shoes or sandals to air your feet. Shoes and hosiery should be changed daily to avoid a build-up of perspiration and bacteria. Hosiery is best washed in natural soap flakes to avoid allergic reactions. A few drops of your chosen Essential Oils added to the rinsing water will act as a natural bactericide.

Aromatherapy Foot Baths

Daily foot care is essential to keep your feet clean and free from bacteria, whether as part of your shower or bath routine or as a foot bath at another point in your day.

Daily Essential Oil Foot Bath Routine

At the beginning of a busy day, a quick footbath (5-10 minutes) using a stimulating blend will energise you for your day ahead. During the day a foot bath can be enjoyed before your next activity, or why not indulge in a hobby as you soak your feet – reading, writing, painting or a handicraft such as tapestry or sewing? A foot bath using relaxing and soothing Essential Oils at the end of the day can be part of letting go and unwinding after a busy day, a sporting activity, tiring journey or a celebratory night on the town.

Procedures For Foot and Leg Care

1. Select the appropriate Essential Oils from the Essential Oil Guide. You might also like to prepare an Aromatherapy Foot Blend ready to use after the foot bath (see page 28).
2. Choose a bowl deep enough to enable your feet to rest flat when filled with enough warm water to cover your ankles.
3. Sit comfortably so that your back is supported and you can relax.
4. Soak your feet for 5 to 10 minutes: a shorter period will not give time for the foot bath to have a physical effect, or for you to experience the healing aromas emotionally and mentally restoring you.
5. Check for any exceptionally dry skin and use a pumice stone to remove it.
6. After bathing, dry your feet thoroughly, particularly between the toes where moisture and bacteria collect. Proceed with the Aromatherapy Foot Massage. Your skin will then be receptive to the oils, which should absorb easily.

Alternating Foot Baths

Alternating foot baths can be used when your circulation is poor. In this case two bowls of water are needed: one as hot as you can manage without scalding yourself, to which you add your Essential Oils; the other as cold as you can tolerate – with ice, if possible, which is pleasant on a hot day.

1. First, place your feet in the hot Essential Oil Foot Bath for two minutes.
2. Alternate with the cold water bath for half a minute. This will stimulate blood flow.
3. Repeat the above six times, finishing with the hot foot bath.

Aromatherapy Foot and Leg Massage

When your feet function well and are in good contact with the ground they can be a great source of vitality. Remember that the body's systems – which include the nerves, blood and lymph – are enclosed within the muscular and skeletal structure reaching from the toes to the head. The state of your feet, therefore, has a bearing on the rest of your health.

An excellent way of taking care of your feet and your entire well-being, an Aromatherapy Foot Massage using carefully selected Essential Oils acts as a preventative measure as well as a treatment. Stimulating and energising massage is helpful at the beginning of the day and will also improve your circulation. At the end of a working day, a soothing massage relaxes and refreshes both mind and body ready for recreation or a restful night's sleep.

Before you begin, check the Cautions Section (page 35) for any reason to avoid massaging your feet. Remove your watch and rings. Check that your hands are clean and your nails are sufficiently short and without jagged edges so as not to dig into your skin. Nails become very strong with regular use of Essential Oils.

Foot and leg massage increases the mobility of your feet, ankles and knees and stimulates the internal organs, the lymph flow and the meridians. These invisible channels of energy, used in Acupuncture, Reflexology and Aromatherapy, follow subtle lines of energy from your feet to your head.

Knees, along with the ankle joints, take the strain of your body and are frequent sites for injury, especially sprains. Knee massage with Aromatherapy eases joint pain and stiffness and helps to release toxins accumulating around the joints that cause water retention around the knees and ankles, making this area puffy and uncomfortable. An Aromatherapist who has also trained in nutrition will be able to recommend a suitable diet, which is low in sugars, fats and acid foods to reduce irritants and promote healing. Rapid changes in weight can be another trigger for problems, as the body has to re-adjust.

How To Make Up An Essential Oil Blend

You can prepare and store several blends of Essential Oils – e.g. relaxing, stimulating and refreshing – in a cool place, but these are best made up as you need them and ideally not stored for longer than a month. Look at the Essential Oil Blends section for 'recipes'.
1. Fill a 10 millilitre bottle with a base oil, such as sweet almond oil, in which to blend the Essential Oils.
2. Choose the Essential Oils for your blend using the Essential Oils Guide and/or the section on Foot and Leg Conditions.
3. To mix the blend, find the maximum number of drops of Essential Oil needed by dividing the number of millilitres in the bottle by two. For example, for a 10 millilitre bottle the maximum is 5 drops of Essential Oil, though you can use fewer than 5 for a more subtle blend.

Aromatherapy Leg Massage

1. Sit comfortably with your back well supported and your legs in a comfortable position. Cleanse your feet and legs using a cotton wool pad with Lavender or Orange Blossom water. This has antiseptic properties as well as being cooling and refreshing.
2. Pour out a little of the Aromatherapy Massage Blend onto the palm of your hand – you can always use more if you need it – and apply a small amount over one of your legs.

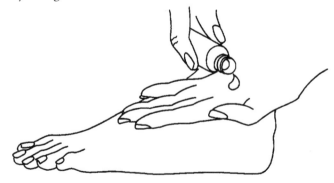

3. Stroke your hands up the length of your leg, moving one hand behind the other. As well as distributing the oil, this stroking or "effleurage" movement relaxes your muscles and eases tension.

4. Firmly stroke or effleurage the front of your leg from the ankle upwards, gently over the knee and up to the top of your leg, skimming down the sides of your leg. Repeat this movement several times until your leg feels warm and relaxed. You cannot overdo this movement.

5. Use the same movement, with your leg bent, up the back of your leg from the top of the heel to the top of your leg.

6. Use your thumb or two fingers to massage all around your kneecap using small, firm circular movements, keeping your hands at the back of your knee for support.

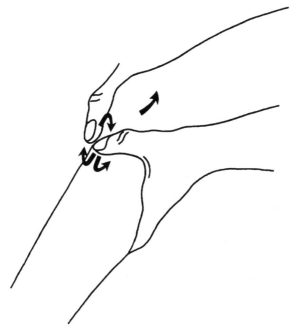

7. Complete your leg massage by effleuraging the whole of your leg, as described above, and continue with the foot massage if required.

Aromatherapy Foot Massage

1. Sit comfortably with your back well supported. Have your leg stretched out, or bent at the knee, or have your foot resting on your thigh, whichever is the most comfortable.

2. If you have not already done so as part of a leg massage, cleanse your feet with a cotton wool pad and Lavender or Orange Blossom water. This has antiseptic properties as well as being cooling and refreshing.

3. Pour out a little of the Aromatherapy Massage Blend onto the palm of your hand – you can always use more if you need it – and apply a small amount to one of your feet.

4. Using both hands, firmly hold your foot and ease out from the centre to the outer edges of the sole of the foot. This gives a nice stretching movement at the end of a tiring day.

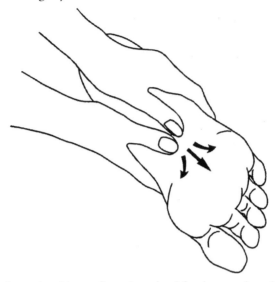

5. Curl your hand into a fist and pummel firmly over the sole of the foot, starting at the toes and working towards the heel.

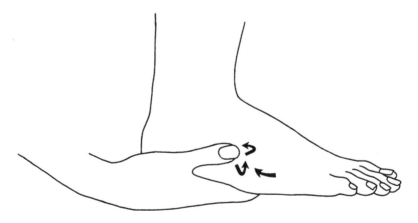

6. Massage in a circular motion around your ankles using technique shown in diagram above, but be gentle in this area, as it relates to the reproductive system.

7. Then move your hands to the outside of your foot and, firmly holding the tops of your feet with your fingers, work the thumb up from your heel to your big toe using the technique shown in the diagram. Use firm pressure, as this stimulates the whole body system and feels good when strong.

8. Holding your big toe with your thumb and another finger, make small circular movements either side of each toe, starting at the base and ending at the tip of each toe.

9. Firmly supporting your foot with one hand, rotate your big toe in a clockwise and an anti-clockwise direction several times, using the thumb and index finger of the other hand. Tension headaches can often be relieved by this movement, which encompasses the point for your head and neck and helps to loosen the muscles in this frequently tight area.

10. Take each toe individually, massaging the sides from the base to the tip, then massaging the ends of your toes, which relate to the sinus points. Follow this by a gentle stretch and tug.

11. Balance the sole of your foot in the palm of your hand and massage firmly between each of the bones on the top of your foot using your thumb in the direction of your ankle. This encourages the lymph to move up through the foot to the legs.

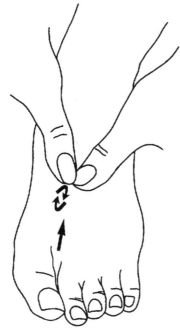

12. Holding your foot firmly, rotate the ankle clockwise two or three times, then anti-clockwise for the same number of times.

13. Slowly flex your foot towards your leg, then extend it so that the toes are pointing away from your leg, relaxing your foot.

14. To complete your foot massage, place your hands either side of your foot and then pause. This promotes a calming sensation which soothes and revitalises your nervous system. Slowly withdraw your hands. Cover your foot and leg with a towel to keep warm.

15. Repeat the above to your other foot, and relax.

Aromatherapy foot massage is not to be confused with Reflexology. Although both work on the whole body, Reflexology divides the body into several zones which each relate to a section on the feet; for example, the zone for the head is found at the top of the feet and that for the reproductive system is found at the ankles. Although there are reflexes throughout the body – the hands, intestines, ears and head are other examples – the most generally used are those on the feet. In Reflexology, the side of the thumb is used in small but definite movements which may be painful over an area of imbalance. These movements are quite different to the massage strokes used in an Aromatherapy Foot Massage.

Essential Oil Baths

Bathing is another effective way to use Essential Oils, as the warm water aids absorption. Oils should be chosen according to the condition to be treated, using the Essential Oil Guide, and varied as indications change.

1. Run a bath of warm water (not hot, or the oils will evaporate too quickly).
2. Add either up to 5 drops of Essential Oil or up to 5 mls. of a blend (this second method is good for sensitive or dry skin and will help preserve a suntan).
3. Agitate the water, then relax for 10-15 minutes minimum.

Compresses

A good method for children. Instructions for the use of first aid compresses should be followed. Disperse 1-2 drops of Essential Oil into the water, lay the material gently on the surface of the water to attract a film of Essential Oil, then place on the affected area in the normal way.

Fragrance

Essential Oils can also be used as mood-enhancing fragrances to supplement foot care.

A wonderful aromatic atmosphere can be produced in a room with an Essential Oil burner by adding up to 5 drops of Essential Oil to the water, which evaporates as it is heated by a nightlight. Sprinkle a few drops of neat Essential Oil onto a cold lightbulb (or use a special attachment) for a similar effect. A saucer of water with a few drops of neat Essential Oil placed on a radiator will act as a vaporiser and humidifier at the same time.

Essential Oils can be made up as a blend and used as you would a perfume. Alternatively, put 1-2 drops of neat Essential Oil onto a handkerchief or tissue and inhale the aroma when required.

CAUTIONS FOR THE USE OF ESSENTIAL OILS

Essential Oils are powerful and should be used with care. For full details, see *Aromatherapy – A Guide to Home Use.*

Remember, **NEVER use Essential Oils internally** and never use undiluted, except where specifically indicated, for Lavender and Tea tree. Keep Essential Oils away from your eyes. Splash your eyes with plenty of water if an accident occurs, and seek medical attention if necessary.

It is generally inadvisable to massage if you have a **medical condition** such as a thyroid problem, varicose veins, heart disease, thrombosis, epilepsy, high blood pressure or diabetes. If in doubt, check with your medical practitioner, who may refer you to a qualified practitioner if appropriate

Do not massage over broken or inflamed skin, recent injuries, broken or fractured bones, sprains or extensive bruising.

Whilst using **Homeopathic preparations** inform your Homeopath if you intend to use Essential oils, as some may nullify the treatment.

If **sensitivity** to an oil is experienced, stop using the oil for 10 days. Dilute to one quarter the original amount and test on a small area of skin before using again. Seek further advice from a qualified Aromatherapist if you continue to experience sensitivity to an Essential Oil. The following oils are best administered by a qualified Aromatherapist: Cinnamon, Clove, Hyssop and Sage.

During **pregnancy** use the Essential Oils in HALF the amount stated. Avoid stimulating and emmenagogic oils, ie Basil, Camphor, Cedarwood, Juniper, Marjoram, Myrrh, Rosemary and Thyme, and only use Fennel and Peppermint after the first 4 months. Massage **babies' and children's** feet with 1 drop of Lavender diluted in 15 mls of sweet almond oil.

10 | Essential Oil Guide for Feet and Legs

BASIL
Ocimum basilicum
Basil will clear your head, promoting strength of mind and clarity when you are feeling jaded from aching legs and feet. It is particularly helpful for ramblers on long treks, who can use one drop of this Essential Oil in a blend for a foot massage en route to promote endurance.

Otherwise best administered by a qualified Aromatherapist.

BERGAMOT
Citrus bergamia
Bergamot is particularly useful for anxiety and stress. When you are feeling stressed, your feet also take the strain as your muscles will be more tense. Use this Essential Oil in your bath for its light, uplifting fragrance.
Cautions: Do not use within three hours of going out in the sun or using a sunbed as pigmentation of the skin may be affected.

BENZOIN
Styrax benzoin
Dry and cracked skin on feet is liable to become a persistent condition if not treated. Benzoin's resinous, penetrating and soothing qualities, when applied on a regular basis, will work on chapped and dry skin as well as blisters. This is particularly useful for conditions which are slow to heal.

BLACK PEPPER
Piper nigrum
When your feet and legs ache and are also cold, Black Pepper, through its action of dilating local blood vessels, encourages your circulation and eases the aches and pains of your muscles. In general, it is useful where you are experiencing a chill after walking or from sitting still for a long time.

CAJUPUT
Melaleuca leucadendron
Cajuput is helpful to change your old habits and to focus on the present. So if the idea of exercise to take care of yourself does not spur you into action, Cajuput can help you focus and change the patterns of the past. For those beginning some gentle exercise subsequent to a respiratory condition, it is wise to continue with this Essential Oil until all the symptoms have fully cleared. If you have not

exercised for a while, your body may begin to clear the toxins in your system, particularly as toxins have a tendency to collect around the joints. As a result, a light fever can develop which Cajuput can address, although medical attention should be sought if this continues.

CAMPHOR
Cinnamomum camphora
Another useful Essential Oil where coldness is experienced. It can be used for muscular aches and pains, rheumatism and sprains. It will also act as an insect repellent if walking in the open air.

CARDAMON
Elettaria cardamomum
A warming Essential Oil which aids the digestive system. Also beneficial for cramps, which can be triggered by a reduction in the electrolytes of the body's fluid. A pinch of salt in a glass of water can be taken at this time prior to a massage which will help restore them.

CEDARWOOD
Juniperus virginiana
Anyone putting off exercise due to asthma, bronchitis or catarrh would be well advised to use Cedarwood, which has a penetrating and healing effect on the respiratory system.

CHAMOMILE ROMAN
Anthemis noblis
This is an excellent anti-inflammatory Essential Oil which is useful for a number of foot and leg conditions. Sensitive and inflamed skin responds to its safe and soothing properties. Joints, sprains and damaged tendons are helped by a compress of Essential Oil of Chamomile, which will also reduce swelling. Do not massage over these areas whilst they are inflamed.

Chilblains, which can often be itchy and burning, can be soothed by gentle Chamomile. Eczema responds well to Chamomile but often requires professional attention to advise on diet and lifestyle. Chamomile will ease nettle rash and allergic reactions, and may be used safely for children in the stated dilutions.

CINNAMON BARK
Cinnamomum zeylanicum
A warming, spicy aroma in a room fragrancer for cold winter evenings, this Essential Oil is otherwise best administered by a qualified Aromatherapist.

CLARY SAGE
Salvia sclarea
Clary Sage is an exceptionally uplifting oil and can often begin to release persistent negative thinking and act as encouragement to seek a healthy, balanced

lifestyle. Physical tiredness and exhaustion may result in lack of care, which reflects in not taking time for exercise or foot care. Lack of sleep may result in physical tiredness, especially if caught in a circle of negative thoughts which may be over-analytical and/or lead to insomnia. This Essential Oil addresses the resulting exhaustion and begins to break the pattern with its warm, nutty, uplifting scent. It may also be used as a muscle relaxant.

CLOVE
Eugenia caryophyllata
A penetrating Essential Oil with medicinal properties to keep airborne infections at bay. This Essential Oil is best administered by a qualified Aromatherapist, other than in a room fragrancer.

CORIANDER
Coriandrum sativum
Like many of the spices and seeds used in eastern cuisine, Coriander is an aid for weak digestion, frequently found with cases of general debility and nervous exhaustion. It encourages the appetite and the return of your strength whilst improving circulation, and helping to release stiffness, weakness and debility. Thus begins the strengthening process to revitalise the mind and body ready for activity.

CYPRESS
Cupressus sempervirens
Derived from the cones of the plant, Cypress works as a tonic and astringent, e.g. as a compress for varicose veins. Useful for bathing and massage where there is excess fluid present, e.g. excessive perspiration, oedema and cellulitis.

EUCALYPTUS
Eucalyptus globulus
Suitable for aching joints, its warming effect is helpful for rheumatoid arthritis, sprains and poor circulation.

FENNEL
Foeniculum vulgare
Indicated for the digestive system, in particular to prevent obesity, Fennel has a normalising effect on the appetite. It can act as a diuretic and is useful in the treatment of cellulitis to release the accumulation of toxins and fluid in the subcutaneous tissue.

FRANKINCENSE
Boswellia thurifera
Excellent to stem the flow of blood, and heal cuts and dry skin. An Essential Oil which has been used since ancient times to promote a feeling of deep well-being and which will encourage a deep and calm sleep after an active day.

GERANIUM
Pelargonium odorantissium
Refreshing and uplifting, Geranium is useful for times when you have been out for a walk or some other exercise or simply want to revitalise yourself at the end of the day. It can be combined with Frankincense to treat excessively dry skin, or with Cedarwood and Citrus Essential Oils for excessively oily skin. Geranium acts as an adrenal cortex stimulant, regulating the hormones.

GINGER
Zingiber officinale
An enticing and stimulating Essential Oil. It is helpful to encourage the body to deal with catarrh, fevers and digestive problems.

GRAPEFRUIT
Citrus paradisi
A tangy, uplifting and refreshing Essential Oil which can be nicely blended with one of the woody Essential Oils, such as Frankincense or Sandalwood.

HYSSOP
Hyssopus officinalis
This Essential Oil is best administered by a qualified Aromatherapist.

JASMINE
Jasminum officinale
One of the most exclusive Essential Oils, Jasmine is useful to address the emotional aspect of physical coldness and tension which influences mental and emotional well-being.

JUNIPER
Juniperus communis
An excellent diuretic and a tonic to stimulate the appetite. Very useful for aching joints and oedema due to its cleansing action on toxins.

LAVENDER
Lavandula officinalis
Often indicated for insomnia, a relaxing bath or a few drops on your pillow will encourage rest and sleep at the end of your day's activities. It is a safe Essential Oil, which will help heal blisters, cuts, bruises and sprains and which will also act as an insect deterrent. It may also be used neat on burns. It is sensible to keep Lavender as part of your First Aid kit.

LEMON
Citrus limonum
Useful for applying onto warts. As a skin tonic it is helpful for cellulite.

LEMONGRASS
Cymbopogon citratus
An ideal insect repellent, it also balances the central nervous system.

MARJORAM
Origanum marjorana
An excellent muscle relaxant, useful after exercise or if experiencing cramping.

MELISSA
Melissa officinalis
A soothing Essential Oil which can be a helpful catalyst in the case of persistent or chronic allergies. It is helpful for skin problems, including eczema, when used in low concentrations.

MYRRH
Commiphora myrrha
Like the other resinous Essential Oils, Myrrh is helpful for cuts or wounds that take a long time to heal. It is also indicated for conditions where there are weepy secretions from the skin. It is a very good pulmonary antiseptic, useful to clear excess mucus.

NEROLI
Citrus bigaradia
Neroli works on the adrenal system, helping to reduce the impact of stress and shock, which affects all of the body systems. Muscles contract ready for action when alerted by stress. Neroli aids the process of relaxation and release of these muscles once the activity is completed.

ORANGE
Citrus aurantium
Like many of the citrus Essential Oils, Orange revitalises tired feet and puts the zest back into your step.

PATCHOULI
Pogostemon patchouli
Useful for cracked skin and weeping sores, it is also helpful as an appetite regulator.

PEPPERMINT
Mentha piperita
An excellent, cooling remedy for hot, tired feet. When used in moderation, i.e. one drop in a blend or in a bath, it alleviates itchy skin.

PINE (SCOTS)
Pinus sylvestris
A good inhalant for general congestion. It also creates an invigorating effect on your muscles, whilst addressing your aches and pains.

ROSE OTTO
Rose centifolia/Rosa damascena
Purifies on emotional and physical levels. Allergies can develop when the immune system is depleted, and the body responds as if it is attacking a foreign object. The Essential Oil of Rose acts as a catalyst to change the body's reaction, enhancing its ability to deal with pollution and strengthening the digestive system.

ROSEMARY
Rosemarinus officinalis
Rosemary has a stimulating effect on the central nervous system. It can be used in blends prior to physical activity as part of the preparation for exercise, to stimulate your circulation and release any muscle tension. After exercise, a bath with Rosemary will help dispel any muscle ache due to the build up of lactic acid in the tissues.

ROSEWOOD
Aniba roseaodora
A soothing and relaxing Essential Oil which helps the body to cope with excess heat and moisture. Also beneficial for cuts, wounds and dry, sensitive skin.

SAGE
Salvia officinalis
This Essential Oil is best administered by a qualified Aromatherapist.

SANDALWOOD
Santalum album
Obtained from the heartwood of the tree, Sandalwood is useful for the throat and chest area. Inhalations and blends will free up congestion and soothe the area if irritated or inflamed. It has a balancing effect on the skin, whether dry or oily.

TEA TREE
Melaleuca alternifolia
This Essential Oil is particularly effective for fungal infections as well as being antibacterial and antiviral. Verrucae and warts can be treated by the application of Tea Tree on a cotton bud to the centre of the wart. Otherwise this Essential Oil should be diluted. Tea Tree can be used on a preventative basis, for example, if you know that you will be walking in places where your feet could contract an infection or be damaged by undergrowth, have a foot bath with Essential Oil of Tea Tree before the expedition. You may also use it neat in emergencies, e.g. for a burn or cut when no bathing facilities are available.

THYME
Thymus vulgaris
Useful as an inhalation if there is respiratory congestion, this Essential Oil is otherwise best administered by a qualified Aromatherapist.

YLANG YLANG
Cananga odorata

Ylang Ylang instils confidence, regulates the breath, and is soothing for the central nervous system.

11 | Essential Oil Blends

You can make up your own blend, as outlined in the Aromatherapeutics section, by checking through the Foot and Leg Conditions and the Essential Oils Guide. Here are a few tried and tested recipes which you can add to 10 millilitres of your chosen base oil.

Enthusiast/Apathy-Buster
2 drops Clary Sage
1 drop Grapefruit or Lemon
1 drop Rosemary

Chilblains/Arthritis
Inflammation present:
2 drops Chamomile
1 drop Juniper

Excessive Perspiration
3 drops Cypress
2 drops Rosewood

Pre-Exerciser/Muscle Activist
2 drops Lemongrass
1 drop Marjoram
2 drops Rosemary

Ramblers' Retreat
1 drop Basil
2 drops Lavender
1 drop Rosemary

Compress/Bruises/Strains
5 drops Lavender

Rashes/Allergies
1 drop Chamomile
2 drops Lavender
1 drop Rose

Poor circulation
2 drops Juniper
1 drop Rosemary

Refresher
2 drops Grapefruit
1 drop Peppermint
2 drops Rosewood

Post-Exerciser/Muscle Relaxant/Aches and Pains
2 drops Cajuput
1 drop Lavender
1 drop Rosemary

Insect Inhibitor
(Use on a tissue or in a blend)
2 drops Eucalyptus
2 drops Lemongrass

Relaxing/Stress Release
2 drops Lavender
1 drop Marjoram
2 drops Neroli

Cellulite Catalyst
1 drop Cypress
1 drop Fennel
1 drop Frankincense
2 drops Lemon
or
2 drops Rosemary
2 drops Juniper

Chills and Coldness
1 drop Black Pepper
or
1 drop Cajuput
1 drop Jasmine
or
1 drop Ginger
1 drop Rosemary

Cuts, Bites, Stings★
1 drop Lavender
or
1 drop Tea-Tree

★ May be applied neat

Dry Skin/Bunions/Corns/Callouses/Sunburn
3 drops Lavender
1 drop Frankincense

Baths and massage

Stimulating/Pick Me Up
1 drop Coriander
2 drop Orange
2 drops Rosemary

War on Warts
1 drop Lemon or
1 drop Tea-Tree
Apply neat on a cotton bud
to centre of wart

Breathe Freely
1 drop Cedarwood
2 drops Juniper
2 drops Sandalwood
or
2 drops Eucalyptus
1 drop Ginger
1 drop Tea Tree

Cramp
1 drop Cardamon
1 drop Marjoram
2 drops Rosemary

Itchy Feet

2 drops Chamomile
1 drop Lavender

12 | Glossary of Terms

Achilles tendon A tendon is the thick, strong, inelastic fibrous tissue that attaches a muscle to a bone. This tendon attaches the soleus and gastrocnemius muscles.

Acupuncture An ancient Chinese method of relieving pain and treating disease. The procedure involves the insertion of special needles into particular parts of the body.

allergies Conditions in which the body reacts with unusual sensitivity to a certain substance or substances, which are normally harmless.

antibodies Defensive substances produced by the body's immune system in the presence of bacteria or toxins.

anti-inflammatory Tending to reduce or prevent inflammation.

arteriosclerosis Degenerative change in the blood circulation system, generally associated with advancing age.

arthritis Inflammatory joint disorder characterised by pain, swelling and restricted movement. It may be the result of degeneration associated with ageing, or symptomatic of disease in younger people.

ATP A chemical compound which when combined with another compound (ADP) in the body cells, releases energy which can be utilised by the body.

ball and socket joint Allows swinging and rotation of limbs.

blood corn Thickening of the skin on or between the toes as a result of friction or pressure caused by tight or ill-fitting shoes. If a corn is present on exposed surfaces, it is hard; if between the toes, it is soft and may become inflamed.

bruises Injuries to the body caused by a fall or blow that breaks blood vessels without breaking the skin.

bursa A sac generally containing a lubricating fluid that reduces friction between a muscle or tendon and a bone.

bursitis Inflammation of a bursa e.g. 'housemaid's knee'.

cartilage Tough connective tissue (gristle), forming part of the skeleton.

cellulite Fatty deposits beneath the skin, forming undesirable dimpling.

circulatory system The network of tubes through which nutrients are supplied to all parts of the body. This network includes the blood vessels, the heart, and the lymphatic system.

coal tar derivatives A series of compounds described as aromatic because of their pungent odour, whose structure takes the form of ring-shaped molecules.

condyloid joint A rounded part that grows out at the end of a bone, articulating with another bone.

contra-indication A sign or symptom suggesting that a certain treatment should be discontinued or avoided.

copper sulphate A poisonous blue crystalline substance produced from copper and used as a dye or a preservative.

cuticle A layer covering the free surface of epithelial cells. It may be horny as in nails, or calcified as in tooth enamel.

dermatitis Inflammation of the skin.

dermis The sensitive layer of skin beneath the epidermis.

diuretic Increases the flow of urine.

effleurage Gentle, stroking movement with the palm of the hands during massage.

emmenagogue Used to bring on menstrual discharge.

epidermis The outer protective layer of the skin that covers the true skin or dermis.

fallen arches These occur when the lower leg muscles become unable to support an arch and the foot becomes weak or flat.

flat-footed see above.

formaldehyde A colourless gas with a sharp, irritating odour. It is used in water solution to disinfect and preserve.

fungal infection Generally caused by microscopic fungi or their spores.

Golfer's Itch Colloquial name for a dry, cracked skin condition, often caused by excessive moisture

hallux valgus Bunion.

hard corn Cone-shaped thickened area of the skin on the toes.

Homeopathy Based on treating like with like. Symptoms are viewed as the body's attempt to overcome an illness. It treats the patient rather than the disease.

inflammation The reaction of living tissues to injury, infection or irritation characterised by heat, redness, swelling, and pain.

lactic acid The acid that causes the souring of mild obtained by the fermentation of lactose (milk sugar) and produced by muscle tissue during exercise.

leucocytes White blood cells, which help protect the body against disease and infection.

ligaments Bands of strong, flexible, white tissue that connect bones or support the organs.

lymphatic system The network of small vessels, resembling blood vessels, by which lymph circulates throughout the body carrying food from the blood to the cells, gathering fats from the small intestines, and carrying waste material to the blood.

matrix The foundation in which tissue is enclosed.

menopause Marks the end of menstruation and reproduction, occurring normally between the ages of 45 and 55.

meridians Subtle energy pathways throughout the body.

meta-aromatherapy Potentially exceptional transformation in conjunction with Aromatherapy.

muscle Body tissue which can be contracted or released in order to move parts of the body,

oedema An abnormal accumulation of watery fluid in the tissues or cavities of the body, often causing visible swelling.

osteo-arthritis Arthritis caused by degeneration of the cartilage of the joints, especially in older people.

psoriasis A chronic inflammatory skin disease characterised by dry, scaling patches and reddened skin.

purine A colourless, crystalline organic fluid relating to uric acid.

Reflexology System of restoring health through compression massage of reflexes on the feet which correspond to the various body organs.

rheumatoid arthritis A chronic and destructive form of joint inflammation. It is characterised by symmetrical swelling and often affects small joints.

ringworm Any one of several contagious skin diseases caused by fungi. One kind appears in the form of ring-shaped patches on the skin. Ringworm of the feet is called Athlete's foot.

soft corn A corn between the toes.

tanning compounds More than one element made up to produce the tanning process in leather.

tarsil area Refers to the bones of the ankle and foot.

toxins Any poison formed by a human or plant as a by-product of its metabolism, especially one of those produced by bacteria.

ulcer An open sore on the skin, or within the body, on a mucous membrane.

varicose vein A vein that is abnormally swollen and twisted. Varicose veins result from increased blood pressure in the veins and damage or absence of the normal valves.

verruca Another name for a wart. Verruca vulgaris, or common wart, is the most frequent type. A wart on the sole of the foot is called a plantar wart.

water retention (oedema) When excess fluid is retained in the body tissues.

BOOKS FROM AMBERWOOD PUBLISHING ARE:

Aromatherapy – A Guide for Home Use by Christine Westwood. All you need to know about essential oils and using them. £1.99.

Aromatherapy for Stress Management by Christine Westwood. Covering the use of essential oils for everyday stress-related problems. £2.99.

Aromatherapy – For Healthy Legs and Feet by Christine Westwood. A comprehensive guide to the use of essential oils for the treatment of legs and feet, including illustrated massage instructions. £2.99.

Plant Medicine – A Guide for Home Use by Charlotte Mitchell MNIMH. Everything you need to know about plants which can be used in home treatments. £2.99.

Woman Medicine – Vitex Agnus Castus by Simon Mills MA, FNIMH. The wonderful story of the herb that has been used for centuries in the treatment of women's problems. £2.99.

Ancient Medicine – Ginkgo Biloba by Dr Desmond Corrigan BSc(Pharms), MA, Phd, FLS, FPSI. Poor memory, ageing and lack of concentration are among the symptoms which the medicine from this fascinating and ancient tree are said to cure. £2.99.

Herbal First Aid by Andrew Chevallier BA, MNIMH. A beautifully clear reference book of natural remedies and general first aid in the home. £2.99.

Indian Medicine – The Immune System by Desmond Corrigan BSc(Pharms), MA, Phd, FLS, FPSI. An intriguing account of the history and science of the plant called Echinacea and its power to influence the immune system. £2.99.

Signs & Symptoms of Vitamin Deficiency by Dr Leonard Mervyn BSc, PhD, C.Chem, FRCS. A home guide for self-diagnosis which explains and assesses Vitamin Therapy for the prevention of a wide variety of diseases and illnesses. £2.99.

Causes & Prevention of Vitamin Deficiency by Dr Leonard Mervyn BSc, PhD, C.Chem, FRCS. A home guide to the Vitamin content of foods and the depletion caused by cooking, storage and processing. It includes advice for those whose needs are increased due to lifestyle, illness etc. £2.99.